The Plant-Based Diet

The Ideal Healthy-Eating Plan to Reach Your Health Goals

Ron Kness

Published by:

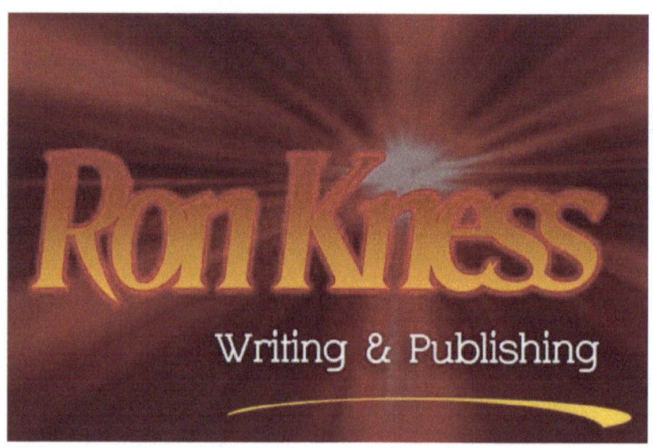

Ron Kness

San Tan Valley, AZ

United States of America

ISBN: 9781689839402

Sneak Peek

The plant-based diet, consisting mainly of vegetables and fruits, has many health advantages over diets that contain meat. For years doctors and dieticians have championed eating a high fiber diet like plant-based to improve health and lose weight, but what's the connection? Studies show time after time that eating a high fiber diet aids in weight loss. However, dropping fat and pounds are only part of the story. Maintaining that weight loss often is more challenging. A high fiber diet can make the difference.

Make Just One Change to Lose Weight and Keep it Off

Many of us have tried several different diets from the Grapefruit diet to Keto to South Beach and more. Usually motivations are to lose weight, but improved cardio health, preventing diabetes or cancer are other health goals. It's no secret that weight loss is hard. Keeping the fat off is often the biggest challenge.

Tracking calories and macronutrient consumption to stay within limits starts to slip. Life pressures from family, friends and work can lead to emotional eating. Before you know it, you've gained 2 pounds, then four and more.

What if there was just one change you could make to help you lose weight and keep it off? According to this study published in the ***Annals of Internal Medicine***, there is! Source: https://annals.org/aim/fullarticle/2118592/weight-loss-diets-focused-1-versus-several-dietary-changes

The study included over 240 people who had conditions like high cholesterol, blood pressure, or blood sugar, risk of diabetes or heart disease. Collectively, these conditions are often referred to as metabolic syndrome. People were divided into two groups to follow one of two programs.

Program 1: American Heart Association Program

People in this group managed several different nutritional elements like limiting sugar, carbohydrates and fats. They were told to eat more plant-based foods including high fiber vegetables and fruits. More fish was also recommended.

Program 2: Just One Thing Program

Participants in this group only had one thing to manage. Increasing the amount of *fiber* eaten each day.

The Results

Weight loss was monitored over 12 months. People in the AHA program lost an average of 3.8 pounds more than the fiber-only people. A few of the fiber-only group did develop diabetes.

What This Means to Dieters

Following a diet for 12 months is a long time. People in both groups were able to lose weight and keep it off.   However, the AHA group had a number of different factors to manage while the other group only had to worry about eating more fiber.

If you hate tracking every single thing you eat, as well as the amount eaten, then the fiber-only concept may be your solution.

Why Fiber Supports Weight Loss and Weight Management

One reason why a high fiber diet has this effect is that it helps you to feel full. When you feel full, you don't have as much hunger and you eat fewer calories overall. In the end, this translates to weight loss.

Foods that are high in fiber also take longer to chew. It generally takes about 20 minutes for your brain to get the signal that your stomach is full. Taking longer to chew your food helps you to get that signal before you overeat. You'll feel more satisfied eating high fiber foods than those that lack it.

How Much Fiber is Enough?

Aim for 35-45 grams of fiber every day to get this benefit. At this level, you'll find losing weight happens more quickly. Continue to eat the same about of fiber after reaching your desired weight to maintain that weight loss.

It's best to get your fiber directly from food rather than taking a fiber supplement. Wouldn't you rather eat food?

The best sources for fiber are whole foods. Increasing the number of fruits and vegetables that you consume will increase your fiber. Other good sources of fiber include beans, whole grains, nuts, and seeds.

Start the Day with a Fiber Fix

In particular, research shows that starting your day with a high fiber breakfast is very beneficial for weight loss. It helps you to kick start your metabolism and fiber allows you to feel full while as you move through the morning tasks.

Most people get far less fiber than they need. There are several things you can do to help increase the fiber in your diet quickly and easily. First, instead of drinking juice in the morning eat the whole fruit. Swap out that glass of orange juice with a fresh orange. If apple juice is your favorite, eat an apple instead.

As for the other meals, always keep fiber food choices available. Some great standbys are broccoli, spinach, Brussel sprouts, carrots, legumes, green beans and lima beans. If is a vegetable, you have a fiber selection.

Eat a bowl of oatmeal in the mornings instead of your daily egg. This will help you to get more fiber without sacrificing protein. Steel cut oats are the best choice. You can also toss out your white sandwich bread and switch to whole wheat or another whole grain.

These simple changes can help you add more and more fiber to your diet. By doing, so you'll find you eat less and have an easier time managing your weight.

This book can show you how to convert to eating a plant-based diet and some of the other healthy advantages to doing so.

Disclaimer

This book details the author's personal experiences with and opinions about the plant-based diet. The author is not a healthcare provider.

The author and publisher are providing this book and its contents on an "as is" basis and make no representations or warranties of any kind with respect to this book or its contents. The author and publisher disclaim all such representations and warranties, including for example warranties of merchantability and healthcare for a particular purpose. In addition, the author and publisher do not represent or warrant that the information accessible via this book is accurate, complete or current.

The statements made about products and services have not been evaluated by the U.S. Food and Drug Administration. They are not intended to diagnose, treat, cure, or prevent any condition or disease. Please consult with your own physician or healthcare specialist regarding the suggestions and recommendations made in this book.

Except as specifically stated in this book, neither the author or publisher, nor any authors, contributors, or other representatives will be liable for damages arising out of or in connection with the use of this book. This is a comprehensive limitation of liability that applies to all damages of any kind, including (without limitation) compensatory; direct, indirect or consequential damages; loss of data, income or profit; loss of or damage to property and claims of third parties.

You understand that this book is not intended as a substitute for consultation with a licensed healthcare practitioner, such as your physician. Before you begin any healthcare program, or change your lifestyle in any way, you will consult your physician or another licensed healthcare practitioner to ensure that you are in good health and that the examples contained in this book will not harm you.

This book provides content related to physical and/or mental health issues. As such, use of this book implies your acceptance of this disclaimer.

Table of Contents

Sneak Peek 3

Disclaimer 6

Introduction 9

    "So, what is the plant-based diet?" 9

    Why it's Easier to Adopt a Plant-Based Diet 10

How the Plant-Based Diet Can Change Your Life 12

    A Real-Life Example 12

    Benefits of a Plant-Based Diet 13

    Proving the Naysayers Wrong... 17

    So, what's next? 19

Making the Change from Steak to Spinach 20

    Easing into It 20

    Planning Your Meals... 21

    Knowing Your Nutrition 22

    Cooking 25

    When to cook and when to go raw 25

    Budgeting 25

    Organic VS Non-Organic 26

    Grocery Shopping 27

Managing Your Weight on a Plant-Based Diet... 29

    The Cardinal Rules 29

    Adapting the Diet to Fat Loss 31

    You'll Lose the Weight Naturally 32

Taking Your Plant-based Healthy-Eating Plan to the Next Level 34

    Juicing 34

    Intermittent Fasting (IF).. 35

Staying Motivated to Succeed 37

Do You Need to Take Supplements? 40

Final Thoughts 42

About the Author 44

Introduction

"The stamina of a camel, the strength of an elephant, and the beauty of a horse are all sustained on a vegetarian diet." - **Old Indian Proverb**

Due to the advent of technology and discoveries in medicine, our life expectancy has increased and more people are living to a ripe old age now than ever before.

In an article done by the BBC in 2018, it was mentioned that the *"average person born in 1960, the earliest year the United Nations began keeping global data, could expect to live to 52.5 years of age. Today, the average is 72."*

While a longer lifespan is definitely something to rejoice over, the hard truth is that obesity has reached epidemic proportions and the statistics for diseases have skyrocketed. So, while we're living longer, we're also sicker now.

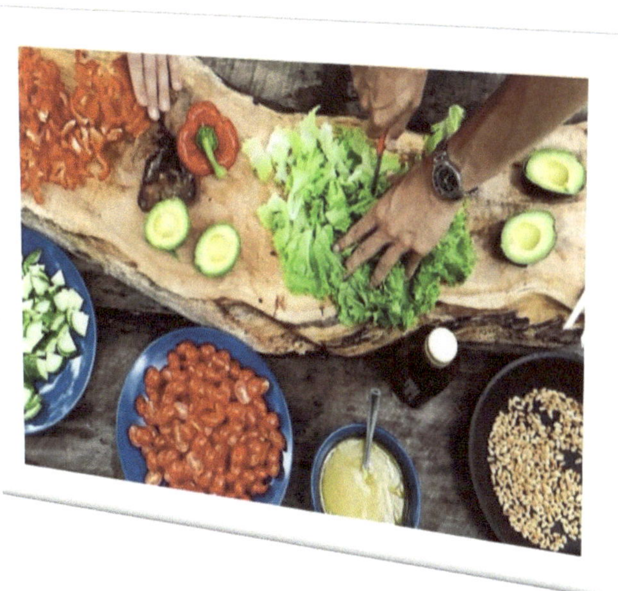

Over the past decade, there has been a slow but unmistakable shift in people's eating habits. We're more health conscious now, and many people realize that 'going green' with their diet will benefit their health.

The plant-based diet has been adopted by millions of people and its popularity shows no signs of waning.

"So, what is the plant-based diet?"

In simple terms, it just means eating more vegetables than you're used to. It means replacing your meat servings with fruit and vegetables whenever you can. That's what makes it a "plant-based" diet.

There are often misconceptions as to what this diet entails. Some confuse it with vegetarianism and others confuse it with veganism. Neither are accurate.

- **Vegetarianism**

This eating philosophy dictates that no meat consumption is allowed. ALL your foods will have to be vegetables and/or fruit. There are different types of vegetarianism and they're named according to the exceptions that people make with the diets.

Those who consume dairy products such as milk and cheese are known as lacto-vegetarians. Those who consume eggs are referred to as ovo-vegetarians. Then we have pescatarians who eat fish and so on.

While these exceptions exist, the cardinal rule is that NO poultry or red meat is allowed in the diet.

- **Veganism**

Veganism is much more extreme and disallows the consumption of any food that is meat or an animal by-product. So, that eliminates dairy products such as milk, cheese, etc. from the diet.

There'll be no consumption of eggs or fish either. The goal of most vegans is to leave as small a carbon footprint on the planet as possible, and to be kind towards animals. By avoiding animal products, they believe that they're saving both the animals and the planet.

Why it's Easier to Adopt a Plant-Based Diet

Most people who adopt the plant-based diet are doing so for health reasons. Very often, their usual diet consists of meat, processed foods, dairy, some vegetables and so on. This is the standard American diet, aptly abbreviated as SAD.

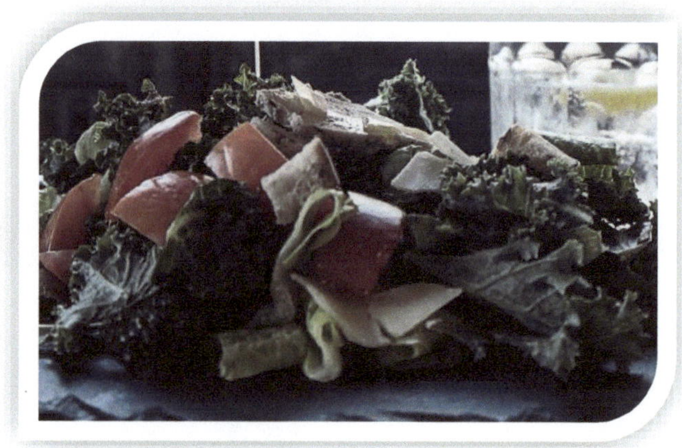

The plant-based diet does NOT eliminate meat. It strives to reduce the consumption of it. This is the KEY DIFFERENCE between a plant-based diet and vegetarianism/veganism.

With the plant-based diet, you get a choice. So, if you're only eating vegetables and fruit for six days a week and decide to have a steak on Sunday, that's perfectly fine.

Or if you have just one serving of meat for lunch, but all your other foods are plant-based, you're still doing great. Compliance with a plant-based diet is much easier than going full vegetarian or vegan.

Now let's see why adopting this rewarding diet will be advantageous to you in ways you can't imagine...

How the Plant-Based Diet Can Change Your Life

"You put a baby in a crib with an apple and a rabbit. If it eats the rabbit and plays with the apple, I'll buy you a new car." - **Harvey Diamond**

Saying that the plant-based diet could change your life is a bold claim… but there's proof to back it up, and the paragraphs below will tell you why the diet will not only change your life, but just may save it too.

There are countless people who have adopted a plant-based diet and never looked back because they saw and felt the difference.

A Real-Life Example

One of the most famous documented cases of switching to a cleaner diet is Joe Cross' 2010 documentary, 'Fat, Sick and Nearly Dead'.

In his show, Joe mentioned how he was obese, in declining health, and on the path to a sickly end. Deciding to take his health into his own hands, Joe went on a vegetable and fruit juicing diet for 60 days and transformed his health.

He reclaimed his health, lost a ton of weight and his results were amazing. You can watch Joe's movie for free here: http://www.rebootwithjoe.com/

While Joe's diet was a vegetarian juicing one and involved no meat, the facts are undeniable. Adding more vegetables and fruit to your diet will result in innumerable benefits.

That's exactly what the plant-based diet hopes to achieve with you. Once you reduce your consumption of meat and processed foods and go for greens on your plate, you'll accrue all the benefits that can be attained from a plant-based diet.

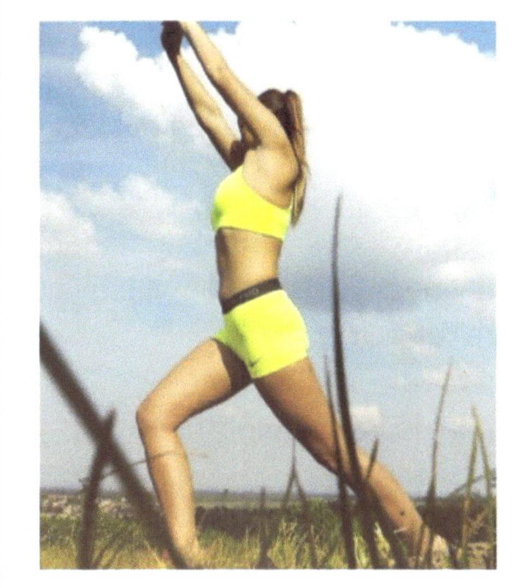

Benefits of a Plant-Based Diet

While the benefits are so numerous that tomes can be written about them, we'll just look at a brief overview of how this diet can work wonders for your health.

- **Increases Longevity**

A plant-based diet could save your life. Just look at what it did for Joe above. If you're on a plant-based diet, it will keep you healthier and allow you to live longer.

- **Eliminates obesity**

When you reduce your intake of processed foods and increase your consumption of vegetables, it's inevitable to lose weight because vegetables contain far fewer calories than the processed foods. Some vegetables are known as negative calorie foods in that it takes more calories to digest them than they contain.

Over and above that, most vegetables are high in fiber which will leave you feeling fuller and more satiated. You'll be less likely to feel hungry two hours after a meal.

This will prevent overeating and lead to better weight management. Vegetables are also more nutrient-dense foods. So, the body will have fewer food cravings.

One reason why you may develop food cravings when on a normal diet is that you may be eating a lot more, but the foods are only high in sugar, salt, starch and additives but lacking in nutrients.

Your body doesn't get the nutrients it truly needs… so it keeps craving more food. It wants the right food… which is the vegetables and fruit that are rich in the micronutrients it needs.

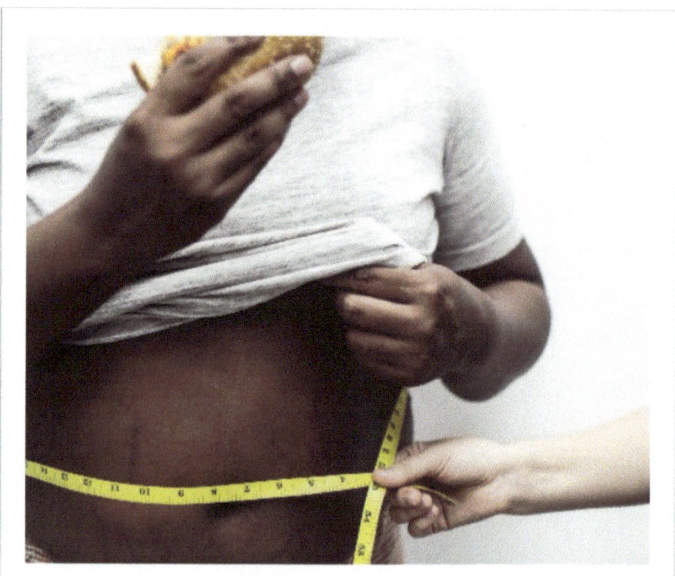

- **Improves skin health**

Your skin is the largest organ in your body. Many people forget this. The condition of your skin is often a reflection of your inner health.

Vegetables will give you all the nutrients you need. You'll notice that your skin is so healthy it 'glows' and the elasticity will improve too. You'll have great skin on a plant-based diet.

- **Reduces Inflammation**

Meat is high in toxins because the poultry and cattle are often given subcutaneous injections to treat maladies in the livestock or they're given growth hormones to speed up growth.

Not much research has been done to show the impact of these growth hormones on humans who consume these meat products, but common sense will indicate that it can't be good to get 'second-hand injections'.

Processed foods such as sausages, spam, etc. are inflammatory to the body too. So are sugary foods and hydrogenated vegetable oils such as canola oil.

By going on a plant-based diet, you'll be drastically reducing your consumption of meat products and processed foods. This will give your body time to heal and your inflammation will subside.

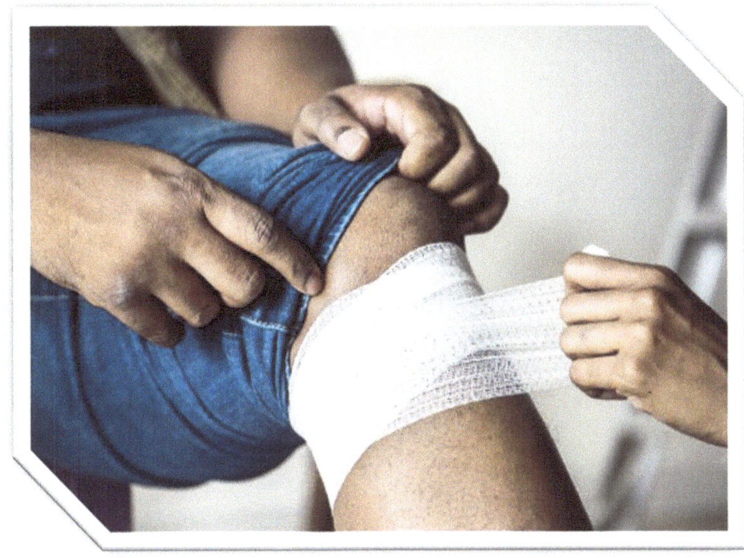

Inflammation is an insidious culprit that sets the stage for serious diseases like stroke, heart disease, autoimmune disorders and so on. A plant-based diet nips this problem in the bud.

- **Prevents cancer and many other diseases**

The antioxidants found in vegetables help to mitigate the problems caused by free radicals in our bodies. The phytonutrients in the plants will boost your immune system and combat viruses that threaten to hold your health hostage.

Tomatoes contain lycopene, which has anti-cancer properties. Ginger is known to shrink tumors and fight cancer too.

Cilantro helps to cleanse the blood by removing mercury and other metals in it. Dill, sage, parsley, basil and rosemary contain anti-inflammatory properties, neutralize carcinogens, are anti-bacterial and help to detox the body.

This is just the tip of the iceberg.

Hypertension, heart disease, digestive problems, arthritis pain and many other health problems can be mitigated or even eliminated with a plant-based diet.

There are a wide variety of vegetables and fruit you can eat, and each of them has their own health boosting benefits. You'll need to do more research on this topic to fully appreciate how powerful they are.

Like the Greek physician, Hippocrates, once said, *"Let food be thy medicine and medicine be thy food."*

He was most definitely referring to vegetables. There were no sodas or burgers back in 460 BC.

- **Boosts your energy**

You'll notice that your energy levels increase when you're on a plant-based diet because your body is much more effective at digesting vegetables and fruit. It doesn't require as much energy. So, you have ample energy to spare.

The fact that your nutrition is better now will also mean that your body is functioning optimally and is healthier and more energetic.

- **Stabilizes blood sugar levels**

A plant-based diet will not spike your blood sugar levels. Unlike starchy carbs or processed foods, vegetables do not affect your insulin levels much.

This is great for those who are in the prediabetes stage. In fact, just by going on a plant-based diet, they'll be able to get out of prediabetes.

Your insulin sensitivity will improve too. This will prevent weight gain and you'll be less likely to get Type-2 diabetes.

It goes without saying that when you adopt a plant-based diet, you'll also need to gradually eliminate your consumption of processed foods and junk food.

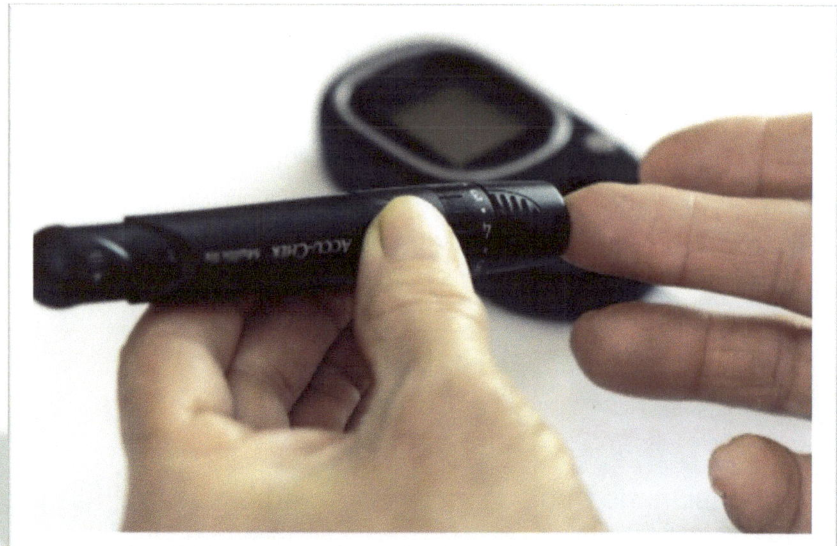

This two-pronged approach will ensure that your efforts yield fruit faster and more effectively. Pun fully intended.

By now you'll realize that you've everything to gain and nothing to lose by adopting a plant-based diet. However, you may have some niggling thoughts at the back of your mind.

These are often due to misconceptions that have been passed off as common truths. Let's look at what the naysayers often mention when you tell them that you're on a plant-based diet…

Proving the Naysayers Wrong

- ***"You won't get enough protein or nutrients…"***

This is probably the most common misconception of the lot. The general belief is that meat makes you strong and has more nutrients. The truth of the matter is that you can get all the protein and nutrients you need from plant sources too.

In fact, plants contain more nutrients than meat and these micronutrients are exactly what the body needs. Vegetables such as kale, broccoli, soya beans, broccoli, edamame, asparagus, lentils and green peas are rich in protein.

You can definitely meet all your protein and nutrient needs from a plant-based diet.

- ***"Tell me why are vegetarians still fat?!!"***

This is a ridiculous assumption because correlation is not causation. The problem here is that many vegetarians believe that they can eat whatever they want because they're not eating meat.

So, they gorge on the processed foods and the high fructose corn syrup in these foods elevates their blood sugar levels which in turn leads to an excess of insulin in their blood… and over time they gain weight and become obese.

It's not the vegetables' fault. It's the processed foods and a lack of control on the vegetarian's part.

- ***"You'll lose muscle and become a wimp!"***

As mentioned earlier, vegetables have enough protein to maintain your muscles. If you're really worried, you can always drink a whey protein shake daily. It's not necessary, but if you're into bodybuilding, the extra protein will help.

As long as you're engaged in regular resistance training and eating a variety of vegetables, your muscles will be just fine.

- ***"Ugh! I don't want to eat cardboard daily."***

This is a worry that plagues many people who plan on giving the plant-based diet a try. They believe that the food will be bland and tasteless. After all, meat does taste better, right?

The truth is that you can whip up vegetarian meals that are tasty and palatable too. With the right recipe book and some practice, you'll discover that you love your vegetables.

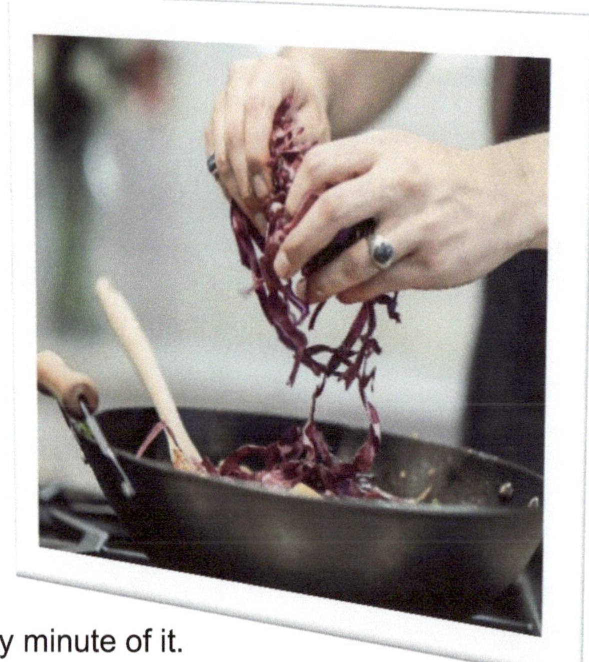

When you go on a plant-based diet, after a while you'll notice that your senses get sharper. Your sense of taste will increase too. Meat dulls the senses, but vegetables waken them up.

So, you'll find that you truly love the taste of plant foods. Many people grow to abhor the smell and taste of meat once they're on a plant-based diet for several months… and finally they become vegetarian and love every minute of it.

- ***"I'm trying to eat… not go bankrupt"***

Organic foods can be expensive, but not all your veggies and fruit need to be organic. In fact, it's better to be on a non-organic plant-based diet than one that has lots of meat and processed foods.

You'll discover that a plant-based diet is actually much cheaper and will be easier on your wallet.

So, what's next?

Now that you're aware of the benefits and the misconceptions, that only leaves one more step to take. If you're ready for it… read on…

Making the Change from Steak to Spinach

"If slaughterhouses had glass walls, everyone would be vegetarian." - **Paul McCartney**

There's no denying that all change is met with opposition, and most likely, this will be no different. Adopting a plant-based diet will mean a shift in your eating habits.

If you love your meat, it's going to be exceptionally tough to reduce your consumption of it. The good news is that it can be done. It's just a matter of inculcating the habit.

Easing into It

There's a saying, "Inch by inch, life's a cinch. Yard by yard, life is hard."

That definitely applies here. When making the switch to a plant-based diet, there will be two factors involved. You'll need to make gradual changes to both.

- **The first one is your meat consumption**.

If you rarely eat vegetables, you can start off by introducing them into your diet. It's common to hear adults say, *"I HATE brussels sprouts!!!"*

Here's a tip – *eat the vegetables you love!*

No one is holding a gun to your head forcing you to gnaw on the vegetables you dislike. Start by eating what you enjoy. There are enough vegetables out there to choose from.

- **The second one is your consumption of processed foods**

Your goal should be to slowly reduce your intake of processed foods such as doughnuts, ice cream, sodas, cookies and so on. These inflammatory foods are detrimental to your health in the long run.

Even a plant-based diet can't undo the havoc that these foods wreak on your body. It's understandable if you love these foods and can't give them up.

What you can do is schedule one cheat day in a week where you indulge in your favorite foods. For the rest of the week, you stay true to the plant-based diet.

- **Making the change**

When making changes to your diet, try to do them gradually. Making sweeping changes overnight will cause your body to rebel. It will develop sugar cravings and you'll feel hunger pangs at odd hours of the night.

Many people try to go cold turkey and clean up their diet radically. Almost all of them fail and give in to temptation sooner or later. The battle is extremely difficult because they're fighting their hormones. Sooner or later, willpower always gives out.

The end result is that they end up binge eating in the middle of the night under the pale glow of the refrigerator light. By the time they're done, they feel physically and mentally drained… and like a failure because they caved in to their baser instincts.

It really doesn't have to be this difficult.

Make small positive changes daily until eating clean and healthy becomes second nature to you. By slowly cutting out the processed foods and increasing the amount of vegetables on your plate, it's just a matter of time before your diet is clean and you're on a plant-based diet.

It may take you a month or two… but it'll be easier and more sustainable in the long run. *Rome wasn't built in a day, but they were laying bricks every hour.*

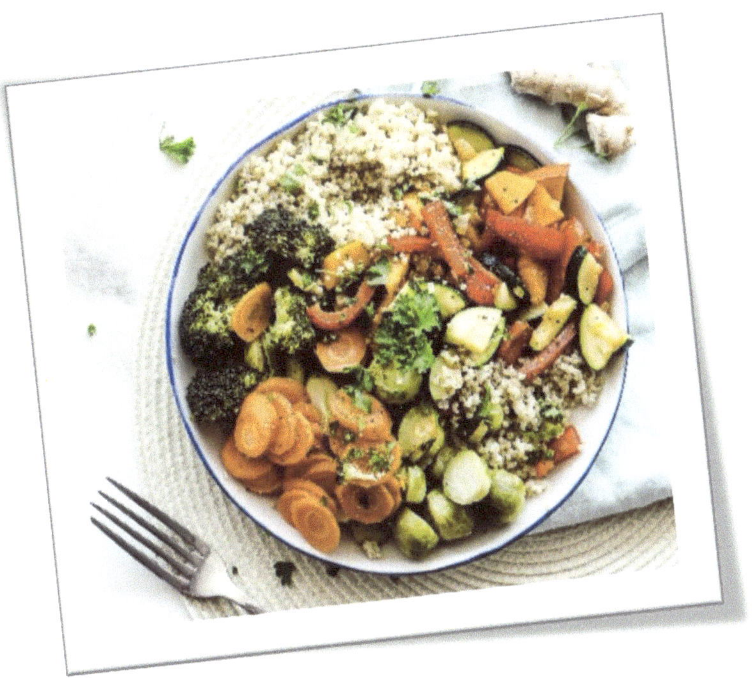

Planning Your Meals

Planning your meals for the week will help you stay on track much more easily. Trying to wing it will only result in failure sooner or later.

Spend 30 minutes on a Sunday deciding what you'll eat the entire week. You may use a recipe book to plan your meals. Take into account your nutrition needs and your schedule.

If you're eating out, will you be at a place that can cater to your dietary needs. If you have a social event on Friday, you may decide to have meat on that day and go with the plant-based meals for the rest of the week.

Always try to be flexible while maintaining a high compliance rate with the diet. Unlike a paleo or vegetarian diet where the guidelines are strict, with the plant-based diet you have a lot of flexibility to work with.

So, plan your meals wisely.

Knowing Your Nutrition

When on a plant-based diet, it's crucial to know your nutrition well. Unlike a standard diet where you eat whatever you want, with a plant-based diet, you need to be more attentive.

Different vegetables and fruit contain different nutrients. If you keep eating the same vegetables daily, you'll only be getting the same nutrients and end up deficient in others.

With a standard diet, since you're eating meat, eggs, processed foods, etc. you're getting your nutrition from different sources. A shortfall in one area is made up for with some other food in another area.

While these nutrients are not the best, you do get a variety.

With a plant-based diet, since it's only vegetables that you're consuming, if you're not eating a variety of plants, you'll be shortchanging yourself.

- **Hire a nutritionist**

This is one of the best investments you can make and it's a one-time fee. Hire a nutritionist and tell them that you're going on a plant-based diet. Ask them to formulate a meal plan for you where you'll get all the vitamins, minerals and macronutrients that you'll need.

A good nutritionist will be able to give you a detailed plan that's easy to follow and may also align with your weight loss or health goals.

- **Study nutrition yourself**

The internet is a storehouse of knowledge. If you do not wish to pay a nutritionist, you can do it on your own.

You'll need to spend a day or two researching and learning what veggies and fruit you need to consume to have a balanced diet.

Below you'll find a handy reference table that will help you out.

What You Need	What to Eat
A	arugula, kale, carrots, turnip greens, collard greens, spinach, Swiss chard, Cabbages, butter, papayas, red bell pepper, zucchini
B1, B2, B6, B12	spinach, bananas, kai lan, broccoli, sunflower seeds, almonds, beans, leafy greens, almonds, coconut milk, cottage cheese, arugula, mushrooms, red bell pepper, zucchini, eggplant
C	oranges, lemons, spinach, limes, zucchini, red bell pepper, eggplant
D	mushrooms, oatmeal, tofu, butter, Swiss cheese
E	spinach, red bell pepper, avocado, pumpkin seeds, mustard greens, green olives
K	arugula, spinach, red bell pepper, eggplant, red onions, bananas, pears, cabbage, kiwi, asparagus, celery
Folate	Spinach, broccoli, chickpeas, asparagus, papaya, oranges, brussels sprouts
Protein	arugula, mushrooms, zucchini, broccoli, kale, cucumbers, cauliflower, spinach, parsley, tomatoes
Fat	avocados, coconut oil, extra virgin olive oil, nuts, seeds
Potassium	mushrooms, red bell pepper, zucchini, eggplant, apricots, lima beans, potatoes
Calcium	arugula, broccoli, artichokes, okra, cabbage, celery, Swiss chard, Brazil nuts, collards
Magnesium	zucchini, eggplant, broccoli, papaya, okra, pumpkin seeds, collard greens, artichokes
Iron	arugula, mushrooms, zucchini, broccoli, kale, brussels sprouts, peas, spinach
Sodium	tomatoes, carrot, spinach, radish, cucumber, bell pepper

Cooking

Cooking your meals at home is an excellent idea. Not only will the meals be healthier because you'll be using the best ingredients, but you'll also be able to eat the vegetables you love without having to settle for whatever they're selling at the diner.

One of the easiest and most advisable ways to get proficient at whipping up appetizing plant-based meals will be to get a recipe book and test out the different recipes within.

Over time you'll discover several dishes that you love and these will be part of your culinary 'repertoire'. Many of these recipe books will be chockful of cooking tips and pointers that you should adhere to.

When to cook and when to go raw

Some vegetables such as white potatoes, asparagus and sweet potatoes should not be eaten raw. Eating them cooked makes them more palatable.

Beans should be boiled. Cruciferous vegetables such as cauliflower, broccoli, brussels sprouts, cabbage, etc. can be eaten raw, but may give some people gas. If that's the case for you, these should be eaten cooked.

Kale shouldn't be cooked because it loses its antioxidant properties and vitamin C. Red peppers should be eaten raw too because cooking adversely affects their vitamin C content.

Some vegetables are better to consume cooked because their health properties are boosted. For example, cooking tomatoes will allow your body to absorb the antioxidant lycopene much more easily. The same applies to carrots which contain beta-carotene which is readily assimilated by the body when it's cooked.

These are just some of the pointers you should be aware of. With a few good recipe books, you'll discover all you need to know about cooking vegetables.

Budgeting

A plant-based diet can be very gentle on your wallet if you know what to do. There is often confusion as to whether you should go organic or stick to the normal product.

It goes without saying that organic foods cost much more. However, not all your foods need to be organic. If your budget is tight, trying to adopt an organic plant-based diet can be burdensome.

The good news is that you don't need to split hairs over this. Going on a plant-based diet is healthy as it is even if the produce you're consuming is not organic.

Organic VS Non-Organic

Organic foods are recommended because people worry about the pesticides and chemical residue leeching into the vegetables and fruit. The rate of absorption differs from crop to crop, so it's difficult to say for sure what the impact will be on your health.

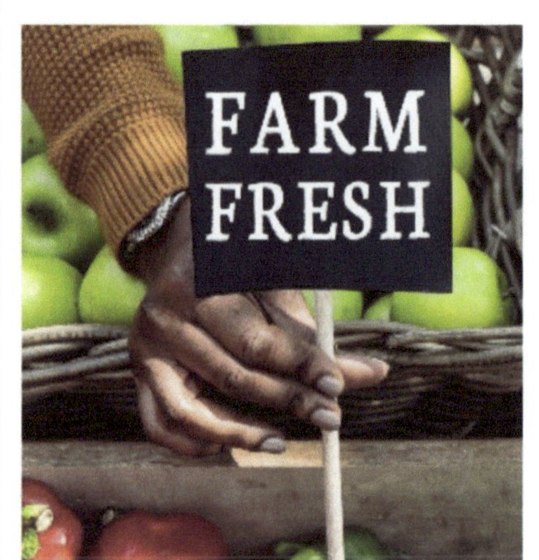

The best way to go about it will be to buy organic vegetables and fruit which are more susceptible to absorption. These are the foods you should focus on when buying organic groceries:

- Apples
- Celery
- Cherry tomatoes
- Collards
- Cucumbers
- Grapes
- Kale
- Nectarines
- Peaches
- Spinach
- Strawberries

Grocery Shopping

There are several ways to cut costs when shopping for groceries. It may not seem like much saving a few cents or a dollar here and there… but in the long run they do add up to a considerable amount. Drops make an ocean.

These are some of the ways you can save money on a plant-based diet:

- **Buy your groceries in bulk**

Some veggies and fruit can last for a while. So, if you can get a discount by ordering more of them, go ahead and get them. Many vegetables will retain their freshness, if refrigerated.

- **Look for deals**

You may wish to shop at your local farmer's market. You could get cheaper prices and even haggle for discounts. Some farmers offer organic produce at a lower price than what you'd get at the supermarket.

You may choose to shop online too. There are instances where you get deals online and the groceries are sent to you the very next day.

- **Couponing**

Coupons/vouchers are another way to save on your grocery bills too.

- **Cook enough food for 2 days**

While this is not a shopping tip per se, it's one that will save you quite a bit of money. When preparing your meals, it's best to cook enough food at one go to last you for two days. You'll realize cost savings when you do this.

Cooking daily is troublesome and you'll be buying your groceries in smaller quantities which makes them more expensive. Buying larger quantities helps you get them at a cheaper price.

By cooking more at once, you'll be killing two birds with one stone. Convenience and cost savings. It's a win-win.

Now that we've established how to get started with a plant-based diet and get your nutrition right, let's use it to achieve the number one goal held by most people on the planet.

Turn to the next chapter to find out what it is…

Managing Your Weight on a Plant-Based Diet

"Nothing will benefit human health and increase the chances for survival of life on Earth as much as the evolution to a vegetarian diet." - **Albert Einstein**

Saying that you'll lose your excess pounds on a plant-based diet would be an understatement. This diet will help you shed your stubborn fat faster than you ever thought possible.

It's more effective than the paleo diet or Atkins diet. The only diet which is more effective for weight loss is the keto diet. Nevertheless, the plant-based diet is more lenient than keto and the results are just as impressive.

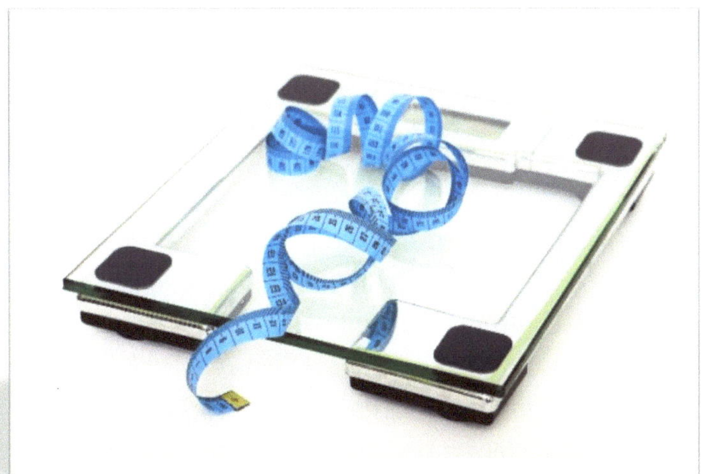

The Cardinal Rules

While the plant-based diet will help you to lose weight, there are a few rules that you must bear in mind.

- **Rule #1 – Aim for a caloric deficit**

The most important rule of weight loss is that you need to be at a caloric deficit. If you're consuming more calories than you expend, no matter which diet you're on, it will be an uphill struggle to see any weight loss.

You can find out your calorie numbers here: https://www.freedieting.com/calorie-calculator

- **Rule #2 – Avoid processed foods**

A plant-based diet is not a license to eat everything else that's not meat. Processed foods will spike your blood sugar levels leading to excess insulin in your blood that's converted and stored as fat.

Adopting a plant-based diet means to greatly reduce your consumption of meat AND processed foods. A plant-based diet is all about clean eating.

- **Rule #3 – Being physically active helps**

While you'll still lose weight whether or not you exercise, by being physically active you'll boost your metabolism and accelerate calorie burning. So, you'll burn more fat with exercise than without.

If you detest the idea of exercise, you can start off small with short daily walks or

engage in physical activities you love. Exercising is not about spending hours on the treadmill or lifting weights and grunting like a gorilla.

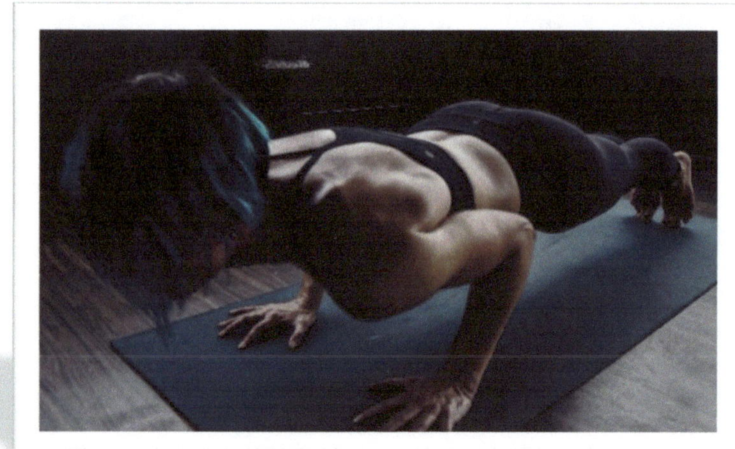

Cycling, swimming, dancing, etc. are all physical activities that raise your heart rate for a while and help you get in shape. Find an activity that holds your interest and do it often.

- **Rule #4 – Plan your work and work your plan**

To lose weight you'll need to plan your meals and your exercise regimen. Even on a plant-based diet, it's easy to exceed your calorie count if you use too much butter with your food or you're consuming white potatoes (which are high in starchy carbs) too often.

Knowing how much you should eat, what meals to eat and when to train will keep you on track to your weight loss goal. While you do not need to obsess over calorie numbers, a ballpark estimate will help you to monitor your eating habits.

Adapting the Diet to Fat Loss

If you're trying to lose weight, it would be a good idea to slant your diet towards weight loss. There are several vegetables that are known as negative calorie foods.

Negative calorie foods

There's no real scientific basis for negative calorie foods, but it's a term that's used in the fitness industry to refer to foods that are either very low in calories or that cause the body to use up more calories digesting and processing the food than the calories the food actually contains. That's why they're called 'negative calorie'.

Foods that fall into this category are:

- Cucumbers
- Broccoli
- Celery
- Tomatoes
- Lettuce
- Apples
- Watermelon
- Oranges
- Chili peppers
- Zucchini
- Cauliflower
- Beets
- Asparagus
- Cabbage
- Apricots
- Grapefruit
- Spinach
- Blackberries
- Radishes
- Green beans

Including more of these negative calorie foods in your diet will help you keep your caloric intake under control.

Another technique will be to consume foods high in fiber. Plants like broccoli, cauliflower, chickpeas, beets, carrots, brussels sprouts, artichokes, apples, pears, kidney beans, lentils, etc. are high in fiber.

These foods will fill up your stomach and leave you feeling full and satiated for hours because they're slow digesting carbs. So, you'll not get hunger pangs and constantly crave food.

Furthermore, these foods are low in calories and will help you maintain your caloric deficit.

Preparation methods

The way you cook your food will also determine how much weight you lose. You'll want to grill or boil your vegetables when possible. If you're drizzling olive oil or coconut oil on your dishes, you should be aware that these are fats and contain more calories.

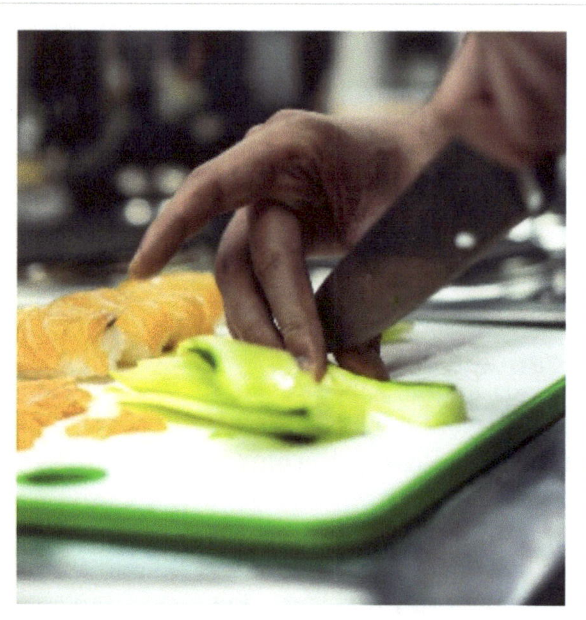

The same applies to fats like butter, ghee, etc. While these are healthy fats, moderation is the key to achieving your fat loss goal.

A balanced diet

Even with a plant-based diet, you'll need to ensure that you're getting a variety of foods. This was mentioned earlier in the book and bears repeating here too. Get a mix of vegetables, seeds, wholegrains and fruit (don't overdo this) in your eating plan.

Hire a nutritionist

Once again, we see this point reappearing. If you can afford a nutritionist, get a qualified one to create a meal plan that's suitable for the plant-based diet. This one-off investment will reap rewards many times over.

You'll Lose the Weight Naturally

The wonderful thing about the plant-based diet is that even without a nutritionist's plan or obsessing over calories, if all you did was to stick to fruit and vegetables and reduced your consumption of meat and processed foods, you'd automatically start losing weight.

It's actually difficult to gain weight with a diet that's rich in vegetables and fruit. You'll realize this once you give it a try.

The excess weight will drop off much faster and you'll be blown away at how easy it really is without you having to struggle as you normally would with a conventional diet.

In the next chapter, we'll look at two different protocols that you can employ to take your plant-based diet to the next level…

Taking Your Plant-based Healthy-Eating Plan to the Next Level

"People eat meat and think they will become strong as an ox, forgetting that the ox eats grass." - **Pino Caruso**

While the plant-based diet is fantastic for your health, there are 2 methods that you can use to get even more benefits from the diet. In this chapter, we'll look at what they are and how they can help you.

Juicing

This is probably the next most logical step when you adopt a plant-based diet. Juicing is much more convenient when you're in a hurry and need a quick meal. A green juice that's rich in antioxidants can be a wonderful breakfast if you want something light.

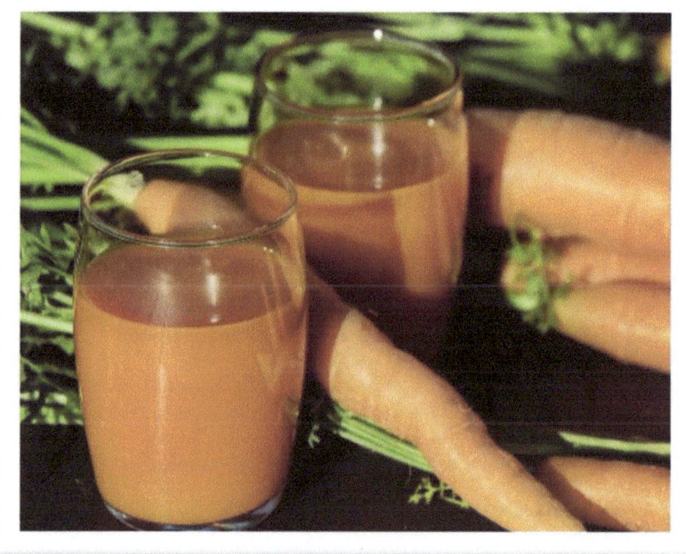

The difference between cooking vegetables and juicing them is that you lose the fiber when you juice the veggies. However, you'll get more nutrients from the juice because the juicer will extract the nutrients from the cellulose in the plants.

Our bodies have a tough time digesting the cellulose and a lot of it gets passed out along with the nutrients. So, juicing once or twice a day will give your body all the micronutrients it craves.

Just like how Joe Cross regained his health with juicing, you too can use it to become healthy. There is a plethora of juicing recipes available online. Red juices, green juices, and purple juices are all made up of different vegetables and fruit.

Have a variety of them in your diet. You'll need to get a good masticating juicer that retains the integrity of the juice. Centrifugal juicers are more affordable, but give off heat which can oxidize the juice and make it unsuitable to store for later.

If your budget is tight, you may go with a centrifugal juicer. Just remember to consume the juice immediately upon juicing.

Intermittent Fasting (IF)

Intermittent fasting is a fantastic protocol that has many health benefits. With the plant-based diet, it's almost a sure thing that you'll lose weight if you do it right.

Many people decide to adopt intermittent fasting for weight loss. However, if you're on a plant-based diet, you'll want to do it for the other health benefits. You've already got weight loss in the bag when you cut out the meat and processed foods.

Let's look at the other health benefits from intermittent fasting:

- Increases mental clarity
- Regulates insulin sensitivity
- Helps prevent cancer
- Boosts your immune system
- Improves heart health
- Wards off neurodegenerative diseases
- Reduces hypertension
- Decreases bad cholesterol levels
- Reduces inflammation and oxidative damage
- Autophagy (cleans and renews damaged cells)

These benefits indicate how potent intermittent fasting can be.

There are many different IF protocols, but you only need to focus on one. That one is the 16/8 protocol. With this method of intermittent fasting, you'll have a 16-hour fasting window and an 8-hour eating window.

During your 8-hour eating window, you'll consume all your calories for the day. During the fasting hours, you'll not consume any calories, but you may drink water.

If you wish to fast for 18 hours and have a 6-hour eating window, that's fine too. The minimum fasting time you should aim for is 16 hours for it to be effective.

Intermittent fasting is not a diet. It's a lifestyle choice and you can stay on it for as long as you want. It's a very healthy way of eating and you'll be able to maintain a lean and healthy body well into your golden years.

Now, if you're feeling overwhelmed and think that it's all too much to handle, do not panic. In the next chapter, we'll look at what you need to do to master it all… and you can do it… if you know how to do it.

Read on …

Staying Motivated to Succeed

"The beef industry has contributed to more American deaths than all the wars of this century, all natural disasters, and all automobile accidents combined. If beef is your idea of "real food for real people" you'd better live real close to a real good hospital." - **Neal Barnard**

The spirit may be willing, but the flesh can definitely be weak. Making the change to a plant-based diet and adopting other practices like juicing and intermittent fasting may seem too much to handle.

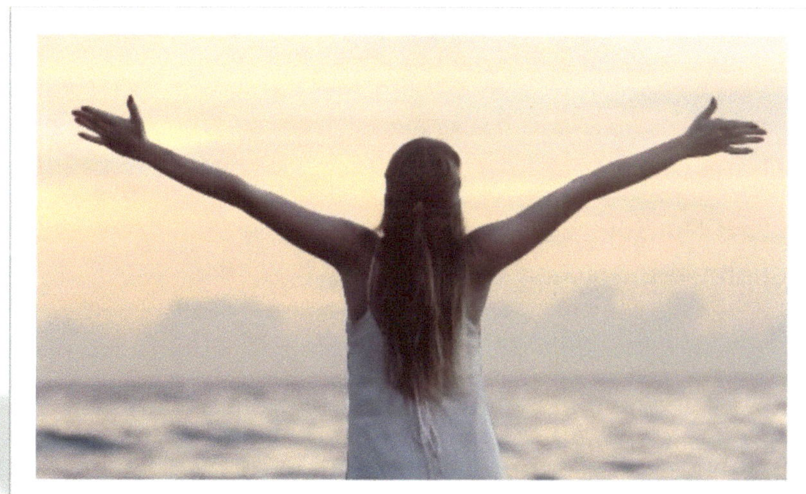

It's easy to get overwhelmed if you look at the big picture. However, you do NOT need to see the entire staircase to take the first step.

- **Micro changes**

In the previous chapter, we talked about planning your meals and working the plan. You were told to take things slowly. What that really means is that you should be making micro changes to your lifestyle daily.

You want to go from having your plate which is plant-deficient to one that's plant-dominant. The best way to do that will be to simply add more vegetables to your meals. You do not have to even reduce your meat consumption.

Just add more veggies. It's as simple as that. This is a micro change.

The next step will be to eat the vegetables first. This will fill up your stomach. Give yourself 5 minutes to rest before eating the remaining food on your plate.

It may seem strange, but it takes a while for your stomach to register that you're full. Over time, add more veggies, reduce your meat portions and increase the waiting duration.

You'll soon realize that by the time you've waited to start eating the meat, you're too full to carry on. Do this often and you'll be on the plant-based diet.

- **Accountability**

Start a food journal where you write down what you were supposed to eat and what you actually ate. Your goal should be a minimum of 85% compliance. If you can achieve this, you're well on your way towards your goal.

Very often, people lose track of what they're doing and where they're going because they have no process in place to track their progress or hold themselves accountable.

Like Bob Proctor said, *"Accountability is the glue that ties commitment to the result."* Be accountable to yourself.

- **Never give in to temptation twice in a row**

Even the best of us cave in to temptation every now and then. If you're trying to avoid junk food or meat but finally give in to your cravings and eat them anyway, do not beat yourself up over it and think you're a failure.

Most people do this and then they throw in the towel and decide it's too much for them to handle. What you should do is acknowledge your mistake and decide not to do it again anytime soon.

Try not to make the same mistake for the next 4 or 5 days. The same applies to any goal you're striving for. If you skip a workout today, never skip the next day.

Once is a slip-up. Twice is a pattern. Next thing you know, you're back to square one and your old bad habits have you in their clutches again.

- **Remembering your why**

Before you get started on the plant-based diet, write down why you wish to start on it. Dig deep until you get to an emotional answer. The truth is always emotional.

Saying you want to get healthy is superficial. Saying you want to be alive long enough to see your kids grow up or you want to spend more time with your spouse is the truth – and it's emotional.

Are you doing it to lose weight so that you're more attractive to the opposite sex?

Do you wish to spare animals the pain of slaughter and just want to do your part because you love them?

Are you sick and tired of being sick and tired and just want the sunlight to break through the gloomy clouds hanging above your head?

What is your why?

Once you discover this, write it down and make a few copies of it. Paste one on your refrigerator door, one next to the mirror in your bathroom and one next to your bed.

Whenever you find yourself losing motivation, read your little 'why note' and remember that if you don't wish to start all over again, don't stop now.

You'll never always be motivated, so you must learn to be disciplined.

Reading your innermost desires will keep you on the narrow path of discipline till your practices become your habits… and once the plant-based diet becomes a habit, you'll probably stick with it for a long time to come.

Do You Need to Take Supplements?

"My body will not be a tomb for other creatures." **- Leonardo Da Vinci**

This is an excellent question and a tricky one to answer. If we were to follow the advice given in this book and you adhere to them, you shouldn't have to consume supplements, right?

Well, it depends.

Modern farming these days is not like the farming of our forefathers. Nowadays, food manufacturing is a billion-dollar business.

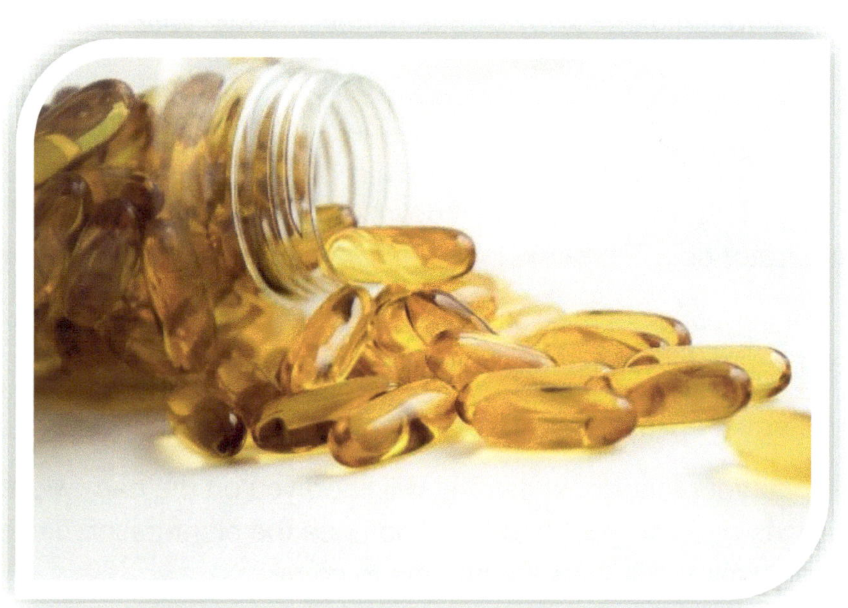

Corners are cut to increase profits and even vegetables and crops are grown in nutrient-depleted soil.

Fertilizers are used to make up the shortfall, but nothing quite beats the natural way. As a result, the plants and fruit we consume may not contain all the nutrients we need.

So, supplements do play a part here. It's best to speak to your doctor regarding this, and he/she will be able to recommend a multivitamin that can pick up the slack if the produce you're consuming is not up to par.

Supplements also allow for more leniency. Getting all the nutrients your body needs by consuming a wide variety of fruit and vegetables can be a chore. Now and then you may slip up.

The supplements will once again help you get what you need. If you're worried that your diet lacks protein, protein shakes are wonderful supplement to give your body the protein it needs.

One vitamin that you should get is vitamin D. If you don't come into contact with much sunlight, it's easy to be deficient in vitamin D… and a plant-based diet may not give you sufficient vitamin D.

It's ideal to consume your vitamin D supplement with a tablespoon of coconut oil and a magnesium supplement. Vitamin D is fat soluble and needs the fat to be absorbed. It also needs magnesium to be metabolized. So, it's best to consume all these at one go.

One vitamin you may wish to consume daily is vitamin C since it can't be stored by the body. While you can get vitamin C from oranges and the vegetables mentioned in the earlier chapter, a vitamin C pill makes it much simpler and gives you your daily requirement in one pill.

Besides these supplements, you may wish to consume others like: garlic oil, fish oil, probiotics, ashwagandha, curcumin, resveratrol, BCAAs, etc.

The supplements mentioned here are just a handful. There are many more that are easier to consume as a pill or powder than to try and get it all from natural plant sources.

While fish oil is not plant-based, it's rich in omega-3 fatty acids that the body needs. The plant-based diet is flexible enough for you to consume a fish oil tablet daily to boost your health. It's an excellent supplement.

At the end of the day, the plant-based diet is supposed to improve your health and well-being. The diet and supplementation are not mutually exclusive.

You can use supplements to bolster the diet and get the best out of both. That's the smart way to do it.

Speak to your doctor and/or do your own research and decide which are the supplements you need. Do note that even with supplements, too much can be a bad thing. So, exercise caution and take a moderate approach to it.

Final Thoughts

If you've made it this far, it's safe to say that you're seriously considering adopting the plant-based diet. This book has given you enough information to take the next step and get started.

Like they say, 'A thousand-mile journey begins with a single step'… and your first step may mean replacing the fried chicken on your plate with a generous serving of stir-fried broccoli.

Or it may mean having tofu instead of steak… or crunchy carrots instead of sausages.

There will be a period of transition and if the journey scares you, make small measurable changes in reasonable time. You'll achieve your goal much more easily if you approach it sensibly.

Focus on getting a variety of plant-based foods in your diet and experiment in the kitchen with different dishes to see which ones make your mouth water. Loving your food is the most important factor to staying on this diet in the long run.

Over a few months, you'll realize that not only have you lost your excess weight, but you feel a renewed sense of energy that was never there before. Your moods are better, your skin looks great and your outlook on life seems to have improved.

It can't all be a coincidence, can it?

Definitely not.

What you're experiencing is the power of the plant-based diet.

On a final note, it's interesting to see that us humans do not have as much acid in our stomachs as carnivores like lions and tigers do. That makes it easy for these animals to digest the meat while humans need to cook the meat to make it edible.

Our digestive tracts are also much longer. A carnivore's intestinal tract is much shorter so that the meat can be passed out before it starts rotting.

We do not have the canines that lions have to tear meat. Our molars are made for grinding, which is what herbivores do.

A sensible person will draw the conclusion that man was meant to survive on a diet based on plants and fruit just based on his physical characteristics.

Give yourself at least six months on the plant-based diet. Once you start seeing and feeling the difference in your health, you may want to stop eating meat altogether. You might have lost the taste for it, or it may even put you off.

This is perfectly normal, and you'll be on the right track. Give the plant-based diet a try today, and you'll never look back.

"A human body in no way resembles those that were born for ravenousness; it hath no hawk's bill, no sharp talon, no roughness of teeth, no such strength of stomach or heat of digestion, as can be sufficient to convert or alter such heavy and fleshy fare. But if you will contend that you were born to an inclination to such food as you have now a mind to eat, do you then yourself kill what you would eat. But do it yourself, without the help of a chopping-knife, mallet or axe, as wolves, bears, and lions do, who kill and eat at once. Rend an ox with thy teeth, worry a hog with thy mouth, tear a lamb or a hare in pieces, and fall on and eat it alive as they do. But if thou had rather stay until what thou eat is to become dead, and if thou art loath to force a soul out of its body, why then dost thou against nature eat an animate thing? There is nobody that is willing to eat even a lifeless and a dead thing even as it is; so they boil it, and roast it, and alter it by fire and medicines, as it were, changing and quenching the slaughtered gore with thousands of sweet sauces, that the palate being thereby deceived may admit of such uncouth fare."

- Plutarch

About the Author

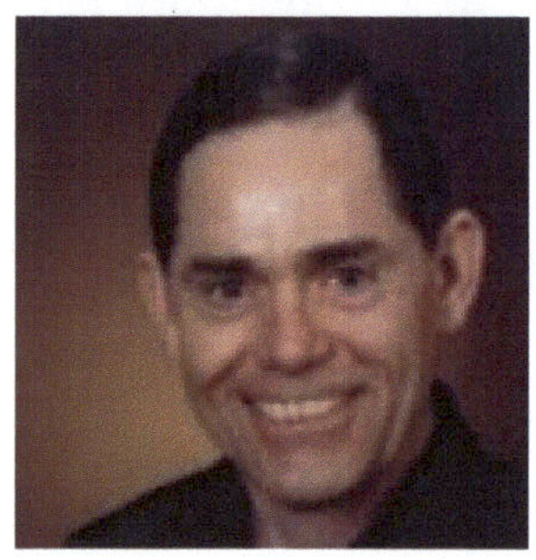

I have published numerous books both digital and printed on Amazon for Kindle and other publishing platforms including Draft2Digital and Lulu.

While most of my books are on health and fitness in general, as I age my topics of interest are geared toward aging baby boomers and the older generation and some of their unique health issues, such as weight gain.

Besides my own writing, I also ghostwrite ebooks, POD books, reports, articles, blogs and do Kindle conversions for clients on a variety of topics.

Today my wife and I are retired from our careers and live in San Tan Valley, AZ. I now write as a retirement business where you'll find me happily sitting in my office typing away on my laptop as I work on my next book or ghostwriting project . . . that is if we are not traveling on a cruise ship - our new-found mode of travel.